Irie Bi Irie Marius
Emery Flavien Akpafi
Kouassi N'guessan

HIV/TB-MR patients on a short course of multidrug-resistant tuberculosis

Irie Bi Irie Marius
Emery Flavien Akpafi
Kouassi N'guessan

HIV/TB-MR patients on a short course of multidrug-resistant tuberculosis

Clinical and microbiological characteristics of patients co-infected with multidrug-resistant tuberculosis: Case of Abidjan

ScienciaScripts

Imprint

Cover image: www.ingimage.com

This book is a translation from the original published under ISBN 978-613-8-47689-4.

Publisher:
Sciencia Scripts
is a trademark of
Dodo Books Indian Ocean Ltd. and OmniScriptum S.R.L publishing group

120 High Road, East Finchley, London, N2 9ED, United Kingdom
Str. Armeneasca 28/1, office 1, Chisinau MD-2012, Republic of Moldova, Europe
Printed at: see last page
ISBN: 978-620-4-17712-0

SUMMARY

ABREVIATON

DNA: Deoxyribonucleic acid

BAAR: Acid-fast Bacillus

BK: Bacillus Koch

CAT: Anti-Tuberculosis Centre

CDT: Centre for Diagnosis and Treatment of Tuberculosis

CeDReS: Centre for Diagnosis and Research on AIDS

MIC: Minimum Inhibitory Concentration

Cfz: Clofazimine

CHU : Centre Hospitalier Universitaire

E: Ethambutol

FQ: Fluoroquinolone

IPCI: Institut Pasteur de Côte d'Ivoire

Km: Kanamycin

Mfx: Moxifloxacin

MIGT: Mycobacterial Growth Indicator Tube

WHO: World Health Organization

PAS: Para aminosalicylic acid

Pto: Prothionamide

AIDS: Acquired Immune Deficiency Syndrome

TAG : Gene Amplification Test

TDO: Directly Observed Treatment

MDR-TB: Multi-Drug Resistant Tuberculosis

RR-TB: Rifampicin-Resistant Tuberculosis

XDR-TB: Extensively Drug Resistant Tuberculosis

Xpert : GeneXpert

Z: Pyrazinamide

INTRODUCTION

Tuberculosis is an infectious disease of humans and animals [18]. Caused by *Mycobacterium tuberculosis* species, it is the second leading cause of death from infectious disease in adults [24]. It has a strong socio-economic determinant and is still increasing almost constantly in the world, particularly in sub-Saharan Africa [16]. The *Directly Observed Treatment Short-course (*DOTS) strategy, launched by the WHO in 1994-1995, was and remains the most cost-effective approach to detect the most contagious cases and to prevent the appearance and spread of drug-resistant bacilli. The global emergence of antibiotic resistance has increased the prevalence of morbidity and mortality from infectious agents [16]. The molecules of the usual therapeutic regimens for clinical categories of active tuberculosis are not spared from this phenomenon, which adds to the already bleak picture of the tuberculosis endemic, especially in developing countries, which concentrate at least 95% of notified cases and 98% of tuberculosis deaths [24]. Sub-Saharan Africa is severely affected by the tuberculosis endemic [22 ; 27]. Indeed, the sustained emergence of drug-resistant species of the *M. tuberculosis* complex, especially multidrug-resistant strains (multidrug-resistant tuberculosis or MDR-TB), remains a current and worrying phenomenon and a health concern in many countries [34]. The problem of resistance to anti-tuberculosis drugs is to some extent a factor in the worsening epidemiological context of tuberculosis after HIV infection [34].

In Côte d'Ivoire, the first drug resistance study conducted in 1995 revealed a multidrug resistance rate of 5.3% in never treated patients [5]. The second study conducted in 2004 after the adoption of a new therapeutic regime in 2002 showed that the prevalence of MDR-

TB in never-treated subjects had decreased to 2.5% [18].

Since the first drug resistance study in 1995 until 2013, patients with multidrug-resistant tuberculosis were put on a 24-month poorly effective therapeutic regimen with many adverse effects [25]. Recent advances observed in the field of molecular biology have allowed the development of efficient and rapid diagnostic tests [1]. In view of the increasing number of patients with multidrug-resistant tuberculosis notified, observational studies have been carried out, particularly in Bangladesh and then in 9 French-speaking African countries, including Ivory Coast [2]. The results and studies on the efficacy and tolerance of the short 9-month regimen have made it possible to revise the recommendations and, since April 2016, to recommend adapting the short 9-month regimen for resource-limited countries.

This short regime, which marks a new era in the management of drug-resistant tuberculosis, was adopted by Côte d'Ivoire and implemented in 2013. It raises a lot of hope for practitioners, patients and their families.

With a view to scaling up the therapeutic management of MDR-TB with this new short regimen in a low-resource environment, the question was to know what are the clinical and microbiological characteristics of HIV-infected patients put on the short regimen (4 Km-Mfx-Pto-H-Cfz-Z-E/ 5 Mfx-Cfz-Z-E) in Côte d'Ivoire

The objective of the study was to describe the clinical and microbiological profiles of MDR-TB/HIV co-infected patients treated with the short 9-month

PART ONE: GENERALITIES

CHAPTER I: MULTIDRUG-RESISTANT TUBERCULOSIS

I.I.- Definitions[38]

Drug-resistant tuberculosis is confirmed by laboratory tests showing that infectious isolates of *Mycobacterium Tuberculosis* grow in vitro in the presence of one or more anti-tuberculous drugs.

1.1.1 By drug susceptibility

Four different categories of drug resistance have been established **[18, 38]:**

- **Single drug resistant tuberculosis**

This is tuberculosis in which the bacilli are resistant to a single first-line antituberculosis antibiotic.

- **Multi-drug resistant tuberculosis (MDR-TB)**

A mycobacterium is said to be multidrug resistant if its profile combines resistance to both rifampicin and isoniazid, regardless of the results for the other antibiotics. Multidrug-resistant bacilli include those with low-level resistance to isoniazid. Resistance to isoniazid is defined by minimum inhibitory concentrations (MICs) greater than or equal to 1 mg/1. Between 0.1 and 1 mg/1, resistance is said to be low-level.

❖ **Extensive second-line drug resistance (XDR-TB)**

The revised 2006 WHO definition defines it as strains of tuberculosis bacilli that are resistant to both isoniazid and rifampicin (i.e. multi-drug resistant) and that are also resistant to any fluoroquinolone and at least one of the second-line injectable drugs amikacin, kanamycin and capreomycin.

❖ **Multidrug-resistant tuberculosis**

It is defined as resistance to more than one first-line antibiotic other than simultaneous resistance to isoniazid and rifampin

1.1.2 according to the therapeutic route [29, 26]

New MDR-TB patients

These are patients with MDR-TB who have never been treated for TB or who have been treated for TB for less than one month.

MDR-TB patients previously treated only with first-line drugs

These are MDR-TB patients who have been treated for a month or more but only with first-line anti-TB drugs.

MDR-TB patients previously treated with second-line drugs

These are MDR-TB patients who have been treated for one month or more with at least one second-line anti-TB drug (with or without first-line drugs).

1.2 TB drug resistance

1.2.1 Type of resistor

There are two types of TB drug resistance: natural or primary resistance and acquired or secondary resistance.

Primary resistance occurs in strains isolated from patients who have never been treated with anti-tuberculosis drugs or who have been treated for less than one month.

Otherwise, the resistance is said to be acquired or secondary, related to selection pressure in connection with inappropriate treatment.

1.2.2 Mechanisms of TB drug resistance

Wild-type bacillary strains, i.e. those that have never been in contact with an anti-tuberculosis drug, are globally susceptible to the products used in the clinic for the treatment of tuberculosis. The development of resistance in these populations results from the combined action of two phenomena: spontaneous mutations in the *Mycobacterium Tuberculosis* chromosome followed by selection of mutants by inadequate chemotherapy **[10].**

1.2.2.1 Spontaneous mutations

Tuberculosis bacilli have the ability to mutate spontaneously, slowly, but continuously into resistant mutant organisms.

The frequency of spontaneous resistance mutations in "wild-type" bacillary populations is minimal and varies among anti-tuberculosis drugs. The much lower frequency (1 in 10^{9}cell divisions) of spontaneous mutations leading to resistance to Rifampicin has been suggested to explain the rarity of mono-resistance to this drug. The probability of a mutation leading to isoniazid resistance is 1 in 10^{6} cell divisions. Therefore, the probability of spontaneous resistance to both isoniazid and rifampicin is the product of the two probabilities, i.e. 1 in 10^{15} cell divisions.

Rifampicin resistance is due to mutations in the *rpoB* gene which account for more than 95% of phenotypic resistance.

1.2.2.2 Selection of resistant mutant germs

A bacterial strain may become clinically resistant as a result of mutant selection. This is due to a variety of causes, of which inadequate anti-tuberculosis treatment plays a large part. In a tuberculosis outbreak, susceptible and naturally resistant bacilli coexist. In the course of inadequate anti-tuberculosis treatment, such as direct or indirect monotherapy, i.e. the use of a single anti-tuberculosis drug or several drugs in insufficient concentrations, the drug-sensitive bacilli are rapidly eliminated and the resistant mutants multiply freely and unhindered. Drug-resistant tuberculosis thus results from the selection of resistant mutants in the bacterial population, following the elimination of the drug-sensitive bacilli by the anti-tuberculosis drugs.

The selection of resistant mutant bacilli by inadequate treatment is well illustrated by the "fall and rise" phenomenon.

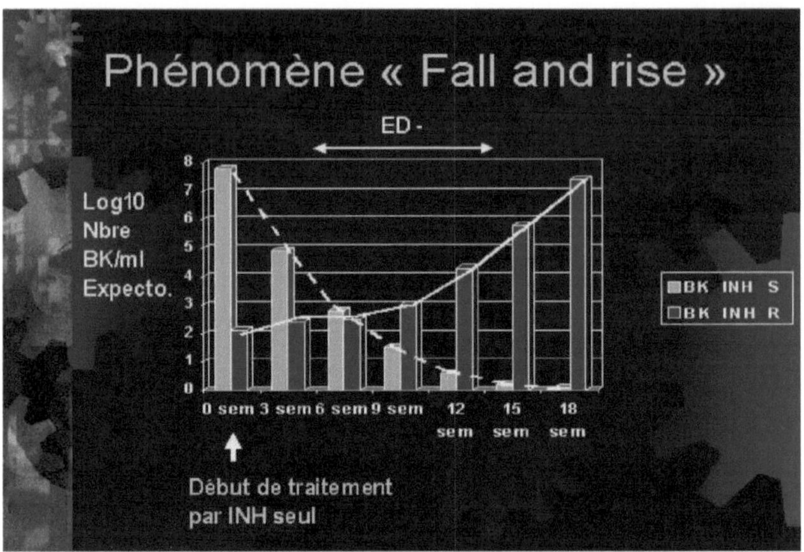

Figure 1: "Fall and rise" phenomenon reflecting the selection of resistant mutant bacilli by inadequate treatments [30].

1.2.2.3 Causes of the development of drug-resistant tuberculosis [29, 26]

Although its causes are microbial, clinical, and programmatic, the development of drug-resistant tuberculosis is essentially a man-made phenomenon.

From a microbiological point of view, this resistance is caused by a genetic mutation that renders a drug ineffective against mutant bacilli.

From a clinical and programmatic perspective, an inappropriate or poorly administered treatment regimen allows the drug-resistant strain to become a dominant strain in a TB-infected patient. The most common causes of inadequate treatment are summarized in Table I.

Continued transmission of drug-resistant strains within populations is also causing new cases of drug-resistant tuberculosis.

Table I: Potential causes of inadequate TB treatment [29]

Domains	Potential causes
Health care providers: Prescribing inappropriate TB treatment regimens	- Inappropriate treatment principles - Non-compliance with treatment principles - No treatment principle - Insufficient staff training - Unattended treatment - Poorly organized or insufficiently funded program
Medication : Inappropriate quality and administration of drugs	- Poor drug quality - Out of stock or discontinuation of drugs - Poor storage conditions for drugs - Inappropriate dosage or combination
Patients : Unsatisfactory patient compliance with medication	- Poor compliance or inadequate directly observed treatment(TDO) - Lack of information - Lack of financial means - Undesirable effects - Social barriers

- Poor drug absorption

- Substance Use Disorders

1.3- Target groups

The consequence of all these factors is certainly irregular or insufficient treatment with the risk of resistance development. These factors have also been used to identify groups of patients most at risk of developing drug-resistant tuberculosis**[29]** :

- Patients who have failed the WHO Category II regimen
- Cases of chronic tuberculosis
- Close contacts of MDR-TB cases
- Patients with WHO Category I treatment failure
- Patients who have failed TB treatment in the private sector
- Patients whose smears remain positive after 2 or 3 months of short chemotherapy
- Patients in a relapse situation or returning after an interruption or withdrawal without recent treatment failure
- Exposure in settings with drug-resistant TB outbreaks or high prevalence of drug-resistant TB
- Residence in areas of high prevalence of drug-resistant TB
- History of use of poor or unknown quality anti-tuberculosis drugs

- Treatment in poorly functioning programs (including those with recent or frequent stock-outs of TB drugs)

- Co-morbid conditions associated with malabsorption or diarrhea causing rapid transit

- HIV in certain settings where the prevalence of HIV infection in the general population is particularly high

1.4- Screening for multidrug-resistant tuberculosis

1.4.1-Elements of suspicion

There are no specific clinical signs of MDR-TB. The suggestive signs are the same as for drug-sensitive TB.

Chronic cough that has been going on for at least three weeks, producing mucous or mucopurulent sputum.

Hemoptysis, most often minimal (blood-streaked sputum), defined as the emission through the mouth during a coughing effort of red, foamy blood from the subglottic airways.

Dyspnea of progressive onset related to extension of parenchymal lesions.

Chest pain that may be related to pleural involvement.

These functional respiratory signs are frequently associated with general signs known as signs of tuberculosis impregnation, which develop progressively

- A fever that is generally low, vesperal or vespero-nightly

- Night sweats

- A significant weight loss
- Asthenia
- Anorexia
- Non-gravidic amenorrhea in women of childbearing age

The diagnosis is made when these signs are associated (recur or persist) in a patient with a history of TB or in one of the target groups most at risk of developing MDR-TB.

1.4.2- Confirmatory test for drug-resistant tuberculosis

The standard bacteriological techniques used include direct microscopic examination of the patient's sputum samples, culturing them to identify the growing mycobacterium, and then determining its susceptibility to the various anti-tuberculosis agents by susceptibility testing **[10]**.

- **Direct microscopic examination**

It allows the examination of smears of the patient's sputum samples, to look for the presence of acid-fast bacilli (AFB) by the ZIELH-NEELSEN method (universally used) or after auramine staining, which allows fluorescent bacilli to be observed in ultraviolet light on a black background. This search for BAARs can be done on the patient's spontaneous sputum, on the gastric tubing liquid collected in the morning before breakfast, which allows the swallowed bronchial secretions to be taken from the stomach during the night. But also on the bronchial aspiration fluid **[8]**.

Microscopic examination does not allow differentiation between *M. Tuberculosis* and other mycobacteria, as acid-fastness and fluorescence are characteristic of all species of the genus

Mycobacterium. On the other hand, more than 10,000 bacilli per ml of pathological product are required for a positive microscopic examination.

Positivity is usually quantified by one to four crosses depending on the number of bacilli observed per microscopic field. Results may be available on the same day. Culture is the most reliable means of establishing the diagnosis.

❖ **Sputum culture**

Culture is used to obtain the strain, identify it and determine its susceptibility to anti-tuberculosis drugs. The LOEWEINSTEIN-JENSEN method of proportions on solid medium with coagulated egg is the reference method. Solid-state susceptibility testing remains essential for the study of the susceptibility of second-line antibiotics, which is the responsibility of highly specialized laboratories. The results of the susceptibility test are obtained only 2 to 3

months after the culture of the samples. The purpose of the susceptibility testing of *Mycobacterium tuberculosis* isolates is to determine the proportion of bacilli resistant to each antibiotic in the bacterial population isolated from the patient.

If this proportion exceeds 1%, the strain is considered resistant to the anti-tuberculosis agent **[10]**.

The methods of culture of *Mycobacterium Tuberculosis* in liquid medium allow to reduce the time of obtaining antibiograms, 8 to 10 days with results comparable to the reference method. The most commonly used systems are the BACTEC method and the MGIT method (Mycobacterial growth indicator tube).

The BACTEC method consists of measuring the production of radioactive carbon dioxide from the use of carbon-14 labelled palmitic acid by growing bacteria. The BACTEC analysis takes an average of 27 days compared to 55 days for the conventional analysis.

The MGIT method highlights the consumption of oxygen in the medium, which is a corollary of bacterial growth, and objectives it either by the appearance of a fluorescence or by that of a coloured precipitate.

The high cost and technical complexity make them difficult to perform routinely in countries with limited resources.

❖ Molecular diagnosis

The culture of Mycobacterium tuberculosis complex remains the reference because it is much more sensitive. It requires appropriate infrastructure to prevent infection of personnel and the spread of TB complex bacilli in the environment (containment level 3) **[3, 23, 29].**

Cultivation is tedious and requires a much longer time frame (4 to 8 weeks). Faster molecular techniques can overcome the slowness of culture. There are several techniques, some of which have been approved by WHO for public health diagnosis of TB and rapid detection of resistance **[4, 37].**

Gene amplification tests (GATs) target a specific DNA fragment whose copy amplification allows the identification and detection of resistance **[19, 29].**

The techniques used (GenExpert, LIPA) allow the identification of mutations in target genes compared to the wild type (i.e. non-mutated reference strain).

The genetic targets most often detected are the rpoB gene, katG and the inhA-mabA promoter region **[23, 29]**.

GenExpert targets rpoB (determination of resistance to Rifampicin). LIPA (Line Probe Assay) targets rpoB, katG, inhA-mabA (determination of resistance to Rifampicin and Isoniazid).

1.5. Epidemiology

The history of TB drug resistance is a problem of recent description, emerging in the last 60 years following the development of TB drugs. During these decades, the problem has been identified locally in certain regions, among patients treated in referral centres in industrialised countries. This was the case with the micro-epidemics of multidrug-resistant tuberculosis that developed in several hospitals in the United States between 1988 and 1991, which mainly affected HIV-infected individuals, as well as some staff members.

With the discovery of rifampicin in 1966, and the expansion of its use between 1970 and 1990, patients with isoniazid-resistant strains of *Mycobacterium tuberculosis* also became resistant to rifampicin. This was the beginning of a progressively increasing problem, reaching epidemic proportions in some parts of the world [7].

Various studies coordinated by the World Health Organization (WHO) and the International Union Against Tuberculosis and Lung Disease (IUATLD) show that the problem of resistant BK strains is ubiquitous worldwide. The results of the third joint WHO/IUATLD survey conducted from 1999 to 2002 in 77 countries worldwide, revealed that the global prevalence of multidrug-resistant tuberculosis among newly treated patients was 1.1% and 7% among previously treated patients.

In 2015, there were an estimated 10.4 million patients with all forms of TB. Of these, 1.2 million had TB-HIV co-infection and the number of deaths was estimated at 400 000. There were an estimated 480,000 new cases of multidrug-resistant TB (MDR-TB) and another 100,000 patients with rifampicin-resistant TB (RR-TB) who were also eligible for treatment of MDR-TB. **[34].**

The majority of MDR-TB cases are recruited from patients already treated for TB, especially those who have failed retreatment, followed by Category **I** treatment failures **[32].**

In Côte d'Ivoire, the drug resistance studies carried out show a decrease in prevalence in 1995 and 2004 respectively, from 5.4% to 2.5%. Despite this downward trend, the number of patients eligible for second-line treatment continues to grow **[9].** The 3 [e]drug resistance survey conducted in Côte d'ivoire 2016-2017 that 4.5% of MDR-TB patients were new cases and 22% were previously treated casesf].

CHAPTER II: MANAGEMENT OF MULTIDRUG-RESISTANT TUBERCULOSIS

II.1 Medical treatment

II.2 Aims of the treatment

The overall objective of TB control is to reduce mortality, morbidity and transmission of the disease until it no longer constitutes a threat to public health.

There are three main goals of TB treatment:

- The rapid and total elimination of all live bacilli present in the lesions, which are sources of human-to-human contamination, in order to prevent the spread of the disease in the population concerned.
- Preventing further selection of resistant mutant bacilli
- The last and by far the most important goal is to heal the sick.

II.3 Drugs used

The drugs used are second-line anti-tuberculosis drugs.

11.2.1. Classification of second-line anti-tuberculosis drugs

The new classification of second-line anti-TB drugs has been reorganized from that of 2011 to reflect the evidence of their efficacy and responsiveness during MDR-TB treatment. There are now 4 groups:

- Groups A, B, and C are the essential (or core) TB drugs

- Group D (with 3 subgroups) consists of non-essential anti-tuberculosis drugs

Table II: Classification of second-line anti-tuberculosis agents [31]

GROUP	DRUGS (Abbreviation)
Group A Fluoroquinolone	Levofloxacin(Lfx) Moxifloxacin (Mfx) Gatifloxacin(Gfx)
Group B Second-Line injectable agents	Streptomycin (S) Kanamycin (Km) Amikacin (Am) Capreomycin (Cm)
Group C Other core second-line agents	Ethionamide (Eto) Clofazimine (Cfz) Linezolid (Lzd) Cycloserine (Cs)
Group D **Add on-agents (no part of the core TB-MR regimen)**	DI: Pyrazinamide(Z) Ethambutol(E) High-dose isoniazid D2: Bedaquiline Delamanid D3 :Amoxicillin/Clavulanate (Amx/Clv)

	Thiacetazone (Thz). Imipenem/Cilastatin (Ipm/Cln) Para-aminosalicylic acid (PAS)

The main second-line anti-tuberculosis drugs with their activity on the main populations of tubercle bacilli, mode of action, dosage and toxicity are listed in Table III.

Table III: Biological activities and toxicities of major second-line anti-tuberculosis drugs line [7]

Antituberculosis	Activity	Dosage	Toxicity
Kanamycin (Km)	Bactericide	15mg/kg/d 1g IM, 7 days a week 10 mg/kg/day in the elderly and in patients with renal insufficiency	Nephrotoxicity, ototoxicity
Capreomycin (Cm)	**Bactericide**	15 mg/kg/d 1g IM, 6 days a week 10 mg/kg/day in the elderly and in patients with renal insufficiency	Nephrotoxicity, ototoxicity
Fluoroquinolones (FQ)	Bactericide for mycobacteria of the	Levofloxacin (Lfx): 750 mg/kg/d Moxifloxacin	Photosensitivity Tendinopathies

	Tuberculosis complex	(Mfx): 400 mg/d Ofloxacin (Ofx): 800 mg/d in 2 doses	Neuropsychic disorders
Prothionamide (Pto)	Bacteriostatic	750 mg/kg/d to lg/d in 2 doses	Hepatotoxicity Digestive disorders
Cycloserine (Cs)	Bacteriostatic	750 mg/kg/d to lg/d in 2 doses	Neuropsychological disorders
Para aminosalicilic acid 11^1-__	Bacteriostatic	4-6g/2 times/day	Digestive disorders, Hypersensitivity
Thioacetazone (T)	Bacteriostatic	3 mg/kg/d	Digestive disorders Skin reactions
Clofazimine (Cfz)	Bacteriostatic	100 mg/d	Skin reactions

11.3.2- Treatment regimens[11,31]

The treatment protocols used for the treatment of multidrug-resistant tuberculosis have two phases:

An initial attack phase and a maintenance phase (continuation phase).

The intensive attack phase is the period during which the injectable agent is used. It is designed to rapidly destroy actively multiplying and persistent bacilli, thereby reducing the duration of the infectious period.

The maintenance phase corresponds to the withdrawal of the injectable drug from the protocol. It helps to eliminate the bacilli that multiply and reduces the number of failures and relapses.

There are two types of therapeutic diets:

- The conventional regimen of at least 20 months duration with an intensive phase of at least 8 months with at least 4 essential drugs and a maintenance phase with at least 3 essential drugs. This conventional regimen can be standardized or individualized

- The short regimen lasts 9 to 12 months with an intensive phase of 4 to 6 months with at least 4 essential drugs and a maintenance phase of 5 months with at least 2 essential drugs.

The so-called short diets are largely standardized and are based on the results of observational studies.

Design of therapeutic regimens

Conventional treatment must include at least 5 second-line anti-TB drugs of opposite efficacy during the intensive phase including:

- Pyrazinamide (Z)
- 4 essential second-line drugs

• A Group A drug

• A Group B drug

• At least two Group C drugs

If the minimum number of drugs of opposite efficacy cannot be reached, in order to reach the 5 we can add :

- A drug from the Dlou group
- A group D2 drug
- Possibility of reinforcing the regimen with high dose INH and/or ethambutol

The 24-month protocol **8ZKmLfxPtoPAS/16ZLfxPtoPAS** is no longer used in Côte d'Ivoire since the advent of the short 9-month regime

The 9-month therapeutic protocol **4KmMfxPtoHCfxEZ/5MfxCfzEZ** is currently used in Côte d'Ivoire since 2013 and following the multicenter observational study conducted in 9 other African countries with the support of the International Union Against Tuberculosis and Lung Disease

Second-line treatment is administered under direct supervision. As treatment of drug-resistant TB is the last option for many patients and the public health consequences of MDR-TB treatment failure can be severe, it is recommended that all patients receiving MDR-TB treatment receive directly observed therapy (DOT).

There is no point in combining two injectable drugs, as there is no gain in efficacy, but cumulative toxicity.

To avoid the risk of selecting cascade resistances, a drug should never be added alone to an ineffective therapeutic protocol.

Table IV: Long 2-line [e]treatment

Product	Weight (in kg)			
	<33	**33-50**	**51-70**	**>70**
Kanamycin	15-20 mg/Kg	500-750 mg	1g	1g
Levofloxacin (250 and 500 mg)	7.5-10mg/Kg	750 mg	750mg	750-1000 mg
Prothionamide (250 mg)	15-20 mg/Kg	500 mg	750 mg	750-1000 mg
PAS (4g bag)	150 mg/Kg	8g	8g	8g
Pyrazinamide (400 mg)	30-40 mg/Kg	1,000- 1,750 mg	1750-2000 mg	2 000-2 500 mg

Table V: Short [e]course of treatment

Product	Weight (in kg)			
	<40	**40-54**	**55-70**	**>70**
Kanamycin	0,5 g	0,750 g	1g	1g
Moxifloxacin (400 mg)	y 2	1	1	1
Prothionamide (250 mg)	2	2	3	4
Isoniazid (300 mg)	1	1,5	2	2
Clofazimine (100 mg)	y 2	1	1	1
Ethambutol (400 mg)	1,5	2	3	3,5
Pyrazinamide (400 mg)	2	3	4	5

11.2. Surgical treatment

The purpose of surgical treatment is to:

- Decrease the bacillary load by ablation of the sanctuary cavities allowing to increase the diffusion of the substances and thus their sterilizing capacity

As a technique we have :

- Surgical removal: elective partial lung resection by lobectomy or WEDGE resection

They are indicated for localized (unilateral) lesions with good cardiorespiratory function

The period indicated is after the conversion of the smears and during the intensive phase

The medical treatment is continued until its end

11.3. Prevention

- Prevention of transmission

- Infection control measures (in health care and other high risk areas for TB transmission)

- Family and friends survey around confirmed cases

- Preventing the emergence of drug-resistant tuberculosis

- Early and correct management of new TPBC cases

- Early and correct management of suspected MDR-TB cases

PART TWO: OUR STUDY

CHAPTER I: MATERIALS AND METHODS

This multicentre, retrospective, descriptive study focused on the clinical and biological data of patients with active multidrug-resistant tuberculosis. It took place from November 11, 2013 to December 31, 2015 in the tuberculosis centres, the pneumo-physiology services, the national tuberculosis reference laboratory, and CEDRES in the Abidjan health district.

Study population

Eligible populations for the study had to have an infecting strain with genotyping results (with at least one mutation in the *rpoB* gene with or without an associated mutation in the *katG* gene, *inhA* or the *inhA-mabA* promoter region), be on the short 9-month regimen (4 KmMfxPtoCfzHEZ/5 MfxCfzEZ) under direct observation, and be infected with HIV.

Prior to inclusion, patients with confirmed MDR-TB/HIV co-infection (GeneXpert, HAIN hybridization test, culture, susceptibility test, sequencing, HIV serology) at the above-mentioned centers and who had given written informed consent were subjected to a standardized interview conducted by the health staff Patient information was recorded in a standardized register. After inclusion, a pre-therapeutic assessment (ECG, audiogram, biochemical, haematological, frontal chest X-ray) was performed. All included patients received the following 9-month protocol (4 KmMfxPtoCfzHEZ/5 MfxCfzEZ) administered under direct supervision for the duration of the treatment. All patients were clinically monitored monthly (weight, adverse events, etc.). Chest X-ray was performed at the beginning and at the end of the treatment.

The bacteriological follow-up of the patients (direct examination for BAARs and culture) was done monthly in the laboratories of CeDReS and IPCI.

The study conducted met the standards of good clinical practice. It was approved by the national ethics committee.

Treatment

The treatment administered to the patients was directly observed. It was administered daily under the supervision of a nurse trained for the study.

Evaluation criteria

Patients declared as treatment failures had a positive culture from the 5th^{e} month of treatment onwards, unless it was an isolated positive culture, i.e. if this culture was preceded by at least one and followed by at least two negative cultures.

Those reported cured after 9 months had a well-conducted treatment according to national recommendations, with no signs of failure, with at least 3 negative cultures taken at minimum 30-day intervals during the intensive phase of the complete treatment.

Data management

Patient data were compiled using Microsoft Excel 2013 software.

The statistical analyses used measures of association

CHAPTER II: RESULTS

1-Description of the population analyzed

The total population eligible for treatment was 132. In this population, 22 patients (17%) had positive HIV status. This latter population constituted our study sample. Thus 13 (59.09%) patients were male and 9 (40.90%) were female. The sex ratio was 1.44.

The age groups between 31-40 and 41-60 years were the most represented with 9 patients per age group or 41%. Patients in the 21-30 age range accounted for 18%.

Prior to the short course of treatment, the treatment relapse category consisted of 6/22 (27.27%) as shown in Table I

Table VI: Initial distribution by clinical category

Clinical categories	Numbers (n=22)
Failure of 1st treatment (El)	**4 (18,18%)**
Reprocessing failure (E2)	**10 (45,45%)**
Relapse from 1st treatment(Rl)	**3 (13,63%)**
Reprocessing fallback(R2)	**3 (13,63%)**
Other(A)	**2 (9,09%)**

2-Prevalence of initial mutations in rpoB gene

The D516V mutation was the most represented with a prevalence of 9/22 (40.90%). A polymorphism at codon 526 was noted with mutations H526D, H526S, H526Y whose rates were respectively 2/22, 1/22, 3/22. All mutations at codon 526 represented 27.27% of the initial mutations. This prevalence is equal to that of the mutation at codon S531L. One patient had a double mutation (4.54%) made by L511P, S522T.

*3-Fate of **HIV/TB-MR co-infected patients***

After the start of treatment, the number of patients who failed was 4 (22%) and those who were cured was 14 (78%)

3-1- Prevalence of mutations

Prevalence of mutations in the rpoB gene among cured patients

Of the 14 cured patients, 6/14 (42.85%) had mutations at codon 516. The prevalences of mutations at codons 526 and 531 were 5/14 (35.71%) and 3/14 (21.42%) respectively.

Prevalence of mutations in the rpoB gene among failures

There were 4 patients who had failed the second[e] line of treatment. Among them, one patient had a double mutation (L511P, S522T) in the *rpoB* gene. The prevalence of S531L and D516V mutations were 2/4 (50%) and 1/4 (25%) respectively.

3-2-Distribution of clinical categories of patients at the end of treatment

Of those cured, 9 patients were initial treatment failures, 3 were relapsed cases and 2 were other categories

Of the patients in 2nd[e] line treatment failure, 2 were in initial treatment failure categories and 2 in initial relapse

4-Association measures

Mutations in rpoB gene and outcome of short 2-line diet[e]

The association between the type of mutations and the outcome of the treatment, allows us to estimate the Odd ratio at 0.81 and the confidence interval at [0.13 ;20.57], See table 2.

Table VII: Measure of association between mutation type and outcome of short diet

Microbiological mechanisms	**From 2nd line short course of treatment Cured**	**Failure**	**Total**
D516V	5	1	6
Other mutations	9	3	12
Total	**14**	**4**	**18**

Clinical categories and outcome of the 2nd line short course

The association between mutation type and treatment outcome allows us to estimate the Odd ratio at 0.27 and the confidence interval at [0.02 ;2.82], See Table VIII.

Table VIII: Measure of association between clinical category and short course **outcome**

Clinical categories	From 2nd line short course of treatment Cured	Failure	Total
Relapse	3	2	5
Other Categories	11	2	13
Total	**14**	**4**	**18**

5-Molecular profiles of clinical isolates: cases of failure

The patients who failed the short course were estimated to be 4/18 (22%). Two of them were ultra-resistant (XDR). Of the 2 XDR patients, 1 had an A1406G mutation in the *rrs* gene, and another had a mutation at D94G in the *gyrA* gene. These patients, in addition to being MDR-TB, secreted strains resistant to injectables and fluoroquinolones.

Among these 4 patients, 1 patient had a mutation in the *embB andpncA* genes, in addition to the *rpoB* and *KatG* genes.

It was noted that the last patient was MDR-TB after treatment.

CHAPTER III: DISCUSSION

The interest of this study was to describe the clinical and microbiological profiles of MDR-TB/HIV co-infected patients treated with the short 9-month MDR-TB regimen.

Out of a population of 132 patients receiving the short second-line regimen[e], 22 MDR-TB/HIV co-infected patients meeting the inclusion criteria of our study were recruited. Our discussion will focus on the mutations in the rpoB gene, the clinical characteristics of these patients and the molecular profile of the patients in treatment failure.

Mutations in rpoB gene

Mutations in the *rpoB* gene occurred in codons 516 (40.90%), 526 (27.27%), 531 (27.27%), L511P, S522T (4.54%) in our study population. The mutation at codon 516 also predominates in patients cured after treatment with a prevalence of 42.85%. Our results differ from those of Lin et al [17] in Taiwan, Ilboudo *et al* in Burkina Faso [13], Sheng *et al* in eastern China [28]. The predominance of codon 516 in cured patients and the double mutation observed in failed patients did not significantly affect the outcome of treatment. Rifampicin resistance is due to a mutation in the protein that inhibits the action of RNA polymerase [24]. RNA polymerase activity is not targeted by short-acting molecules. This could explain why mutations do not appear to be a factor in failure of this regimen.

Clinical characteristics

Patients were classified into clinical categories on the basis of previous treatment with anti-tuberculosis drugs. The duration of previous treatment did not put the patients at risk of treatment failure. This success could be explained by the fact that short course drugs have a high efficacy and good pulmonary diffusion in co-infected patients. The DOTS strategy would be an adequate solution to the therapeutic success of the short course of treatment[e]

Molecular profile of patients in therapeutic failure.

At the end of the treatment, 4 patients were in therapeutic failure of which 2 XDR, in spite of the effectiveness of the treatment and the strategy of the directly observed treatment. These patients would probably have escaped therapeutic control. One might ask, did these patients really follow the DOTS strategy during treatment? Were they diagnosed in time? The probable extent of the very large lesions, due to a probable late diagnosis in these patients could have been the cause of their failure.

CONCLUSION

MDR-TB/HIV co-infection is emerging in our tropics. At the end of this study, which aimed to describe the clinical and microbiological profiles of 22 patients co-infected with MDR-TB/HIV treated with the short 9-month regimen, it appeared that the D516V mutation was predominant, followed by a polymorphism at codon 526, a doubly mutated patient was cured in 78% of the co-infected patients, and that 6 of the XDR patients had relapsed on treatment, and that there were 2 XDRs among the patients who had failed on the treatment. No clinical and biological factor would be likely to lead to a therapeutic failure of the short course in these patients. The implementation of the short course of treatment of 2^{e}lines constitutes a hope in the management of MDR-TB in general and more particularly in the co-infection MDR-TB/HIV. The fight against this co-infection should be increased, as it would be a ray of hope for the populations.

BIBLIOGRAPHIC REFERENCES

1. **Adegbele J.A.** Performance of three diagnostic tools for pulmonary tuberculosis in Abidjan : Thesis Med ,2015. n°5822

2. **Aung K.J.M, Deun V, Declercq E, Sarker M.R, Das P.K, Hossain M.A, et al.** Success of a 9-month protocol for treatment of multidrug-resistant tuberculosis in 500 consecutive patients in Bangladesh, INT J tuberc lung dis 2014 18(10):1180-7

3. **Bonnet M.** New diagnostic tests for tuberculosis disease: from theory to practice in the South. Tuberculosis and Mycobacterium series. *Rev MalResp 2011; 28(10): 131021.*

4. **Borell S, Gagneux S.** Contagiousness, reproductive capacity and evolution of drug-resistant Mycobacterium Tuberculosis. *Int J Tuberc Lung Dis 2009; 12(12): 1456-66*

5. **Cambau E.** Diagnostic tools for resistance: current practices and perspectives.2013.Accessed on 31/03/2017 from invs.santépubliquefrance.fr

6. **Caminero JA.** Multidrug-resistant tuberculosis: epidemiology, risk factor and case finding. *Int J Tuberc Lung Dis 2010; 14(4): 382-90.*

7. **Dao Y.** Therapeutic follow-up of isoniazid in patients with a first episode of microcopy-positive pulmonary tuberculosis in the Pneumophthisiology Department of Treichville University Hospital. *Thesis of medicine Abidjan 2014;*

8. **Doris Hillemann, Tanja Kubica, Sabine Rûsch-Gerdes, and Stefan** Niemann Disequilibrium in Distribution of Resistance Mutations among Mycobacterium tuberculosis Beijing and Non-Beijing Strains Isolated from Patients in Germany. Antimicrobial Agents and Chemotherapy. 2005, 49(3): 1229-31

9. Dosso M, Bonard D, Msellati P, Bamba A, Doulhourou. Primary resistance to anti-tuberculosis drugs: a national survey conducted in Côte d'Ivoire in 1995-1996, 1999. Intj tuberc lung dis 3 (9): 805-9

10. Respiratory Disease Fund. Diagnosis and treatment of tuberculosis, practical manual, recommendations for the medical profession. *FARESasbl 2010.*

www.fares.be/recommandationsTBC2010.pdf

11. Frechet JM, Metivier N. Resistant tuberculosis. EMC (ElsevierMasson **SAS,** Paris). Pneumology 2009, 6-019-A35

12. Guessennd K. N.Bacterial resistance to antibiotics in Africa.2013.Document accessed on 15/04/2017 onhttp//www.assiteb-biorif.com

13. Ilboudo Désiré. Molecular diagnosis by real time PCR of *Mycobacterium tuberculosis* complex resistant to isoniazid and rifampicin. Dissertation from the laboratory of molecular biology and molecular genetics (Labiogene), Ouagadougou, 2013.

14. Jun Y,Wei S, Jingping X, Yao L, Erliang Z, and Honghai W. Mutations in the *rpoB* Gene of Multidrug-Resistant Mycobacterium tuberculosis Isolates from China. Journal of Clinical Microbiology, 2003; 41(5), 2209-12

15. Kouassi B, Horo K, N'DoubaK.A, Koffi N,Ngom A, Bangui A, Dosso M.Epidemiological and microbiological profile of tuberculosis patients in failure or relapse situation in Abidjan. Bull Soc Pathol Exot, 2004, 97, 5, 336-337

16. Lavender V. new microbiological tools for tuberculosis: what perspectives. La Lettre de l'Infectiologue.January-February 2012. Volume 27 -n° 1

17. LIN, Y. H, TAI, C. H, LI,C.R, LIN,C.F, SHI,Z.Y. (2012). Resistance profiles and *rpoB* gene mutationofMycobacteriom tuberculosis isolates in Taiwan./Microbiol Immunol

18. LoBue P. A, Enarson D. A, Thoen. C. O. Tuberculosis: a resurgent condition in animals and humans; 2010. Intj tuberc lung dis ,2010 ;14(9):1075-8

19. Nguessan K, Ouassa T, Assi JS, Tehe A, Assande JM, Guei A et al. Molecular detection of rifampicin and isoniazid among patients eligible for retreatment regimen in Côte d'Ivoire in 2012. *Advances in Infectious Diseases 2013; 3: 65-70.*

20. WHO. Geneva: WHO; World TB Control Report. 2010.

21. WHO. Global TB Control Programme. Planning for the implementation of new diagnostics. Workshop on the development of national strategic plans for TB control. 2014, Rabat. Morocco

22. WHO-Geneva. Guidelines for tuberculosis programmes for the management of drug-resistant tuberculosis. Emergency update for 2008. *Geneva, Switzerland: WHO 2009; 276p.*

23. PAI M, MINION J, SOHN H et al. Novel and improved technologies for tuberculosis diagnosis: progress and challenges. *Clin Chest Med 2009; 30: 701-16.*

24. Burkina Faso National Tuberculosis Control Programme. Technical guide for the management of drug-resistant tuberculosis cases in Burkina Faso. Edition 2009. 9-13p

25. National Tuberculosis Control Programme of Cote d'Ivoire. National guidelines for the therapeutic management of tuberculosis. February 2011 edition

26. National Tuberculosis Control Programme of Côte d'Ivoire. National guidelines for the management of drug-resistant tuberculosis in Côte d'Ivoire. *Edition 2013.*

27. **Raviglione M. C, O'Brien. R. J.** Harrison's principles ofinternal medicine. 17th Edition. USA: The McGraw-Hill Companies; 2008. Tuberculosis.

28. **Sheng J, sheng G, Yu H, Cao H, Lu Y.** Charsterization of *rpoB* mutations associated with rifam resistance in Mycobacterium tuberculosis from eastern China. Journal of Applied Microbiology 105(2008)904-11

29. **VAN DEUN A, MARTIN A, PALOMINO JC.** Diagnosis of drug-resistant tuberculosis: reliability and speed of detection. *Int J Tuberc Lung Dis 2010; 14(2): 131-40.*

30. **Van Vooren JP**. Multidrug-resistant tuberculosis. Infectious pathology seminar February 28, 2002. Retrieved from www.seminfect.be/dias...28,../tsdl021.ht... on 04-11-2014

31. **WHO.** WHO treatment guidelines for drug-resistant tuberculosis. 2016 update.

32. www.who.int//tb/publications

33. **WHO.** Anti-tuberculosis drug-resistant in the world, fourth global report 2008. www.who.int//tb/publications

34. **World health organization .** Guidelines for treatement of tuberculosis. WHO/HTM/TB/2009.420, Geneva, Switzerland

35. **World health organization.** Multidrug-resistanttuberculosis. October 2016

36. **World Health Organisation.What is DOTS?** A Guide to Understanding the WHO-recommended TB Control Strategy Known as DOTS. WHO/CDS/CPC/TB/99.270, World Health Organization, Geneva, Switzerland.

37. World Health Organization. THE STOP TB STRATEGY: Building on and enhancing DOTS to meet the TB-related Millennium Development Goals.WHO/HTM/TB/2006.368. World Health Organization, Geneva, Switzerland.

38. WHO. Policy statement: Molecular line probe assays for rapid screening of patients at risk of multidrug-resistant tuberculosis (MDR-TB). WHO, Geneva 2009 www.who.int/tb/line probe assays/en/

39.. WHO. Guideline for the programmatic management of drug-resistant tuberculosis. 2011 update. *WHO/HTM/2011.6*

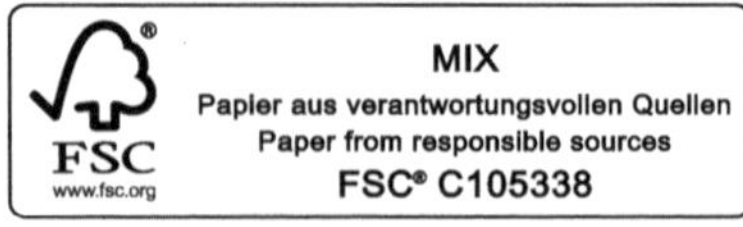

Printed by Books on Demand GmbH, Norderstedt / Germany